THE LITTLE BOOK OF
HOMEOPATHY

For Aundie and Occy

THE LITTLE BOOK OF

HOMEOPATHY

Practical tips for effective
self-treatment

SVEN SOMMER

VERMILION
LONDON

1 3 5 7 9 10 8 6 4 2

First published in the United Kingdom in 2001 by Vermilion,
an imprint of Ebury Press, Random House,
20 Vauxhall Bridge Road, London SW1V 2SA
www.randomhouse.co.uk

Random House Australia (Pty) Limited
20 Alfred Street, Milsons Point, Sydney, New South Wales
2061, Australia

Random House New Zealand Limited
18 Poland Road, Glenfield, Auckland 10, New Zealand

Random House South Africa (Pty) Limited
Endulini, 5a Jubilee Road, Parktown 2193, South Africa

The Random House Group Limited Reg. No. 954009

Papers used by Vermilion are natural, recyclable products made
from woodgrown in sustainable forests.

Printed and bound in Denmark by Nørhaven A/S, Viborg

A CIP catalogue record for this book is available from the
British Library.

ISBN 0 09 185705 8

CONTENTS

PART I

PART 2

PART 3

DEAR READER

Welcome to *The Little Book of Homeopathy*: a concise but comprehensive introduction to the magical world of the minimum dose. This was how Goethe, the great German poet, once described homeopathy. With this self-help booklet you can experience first hand a gentle but effective way of healing. Free from any side effects, homeopathy is perfectly suited to self-treatment. Everyday, minor complaints can be safely dealt with at home.

The Little Book of Homeopathy has been specifically designed with this in mind: it will slip easily into your pocket and fit neatly into a homeopathic kit (see page 24). This handy combination of remedy-kit and mini-guide can be kept within easy reach at home or on holiday.

Part 1 of this guide should be read carefully. It explains how homeopathic treatment works and tells you how to use the remedies safely. Part 2 lists a number of common complaints in alphabetical order together with the appropriate remedies. This is followed by a section on homeopathic treatment specific to children and babies. Finally, in Part 3, each of the remedies is described in more detail, together with relevant symptoms and complaints for which they are recommended.

Sven Sommer

PART I

WHAT IS HOMEOPATHY?

Homeopathy is an effective complementary treatment based upon a holistic approach to health. It looks at the whole person and the root cause of the illness, not just at the specific symptoms. Homeopathy has one objective: to stimulate the body's own defence mechanism or immune system. By strengthening our own natural healing forces, we can overcome illness and enjoy good health.

Homeopathy is based on the following principle: a substance taken in a toxic dose will produce certain specific symptoms of illness in a healthy person. That same substance taken in a minimum dose can cure a sick person with similar symptoms. The diluted dose stimulates the body's own defence system and initiates the process of self-healing. Samuel Hahnemann, founder of homeopathy, described this as the law of similarities or the cure of 'like with like'. Such a mechanism is already known in the field of immunisation. For example, the diluted cowpox serum was used successfully in immunisation against smallpox. A homeopathic treatment for symptoms similar to those of a bee-sting (pale-red swelling, stinging pain) would therefore be the preparation of 'Apis', the bee. It would alleviate the condition.

Homeopathy is scientifically based and developed through controlled experimental testing. Human volunteers are used for this research; there is no animal testing! Before antibiotics were invented, homeopathy was accepted as a conventional form of medical treatment. Today, increasing numbers of bacteria are becoming resistant to antibiotics and doctors are more reluctant to prescribe them. For many common viral illnesses, there is little more that mainstream medicine can offer other than rest and aspirin. Homeopathy, on the other hand, offers a wide range of remedies which are extremely effective in the treatment of such cases.

For this reason, increasing numbers of GPs are now reverting to homeopathic medicine. In chronic conditions, homeopathy is also known to produce positive results. Hahnemann's discovery may once again prove to be an important part of mainstream medicine.

The treatment

When treating a complaint, the homeopath selects the substance which has the potential to provoke similar symptoms. This substance, highly diluted and specifically prepared, boosts our defence mechanisms in their battle against the illness and stimulates the healing process. In this way homeopathy strengthens the immune system and has a profound positive effect on our health.

While the homeopath searches for the most similar remedy, she/he has to pay attention to all the patient's symptoms and consider the whole picture of their physical and emotional condition. The homeopath will observe, examine and interview the patient with close attention to detail. Enquiries will be made as to when the symptoms first appeared, the possible cause, and what improves or aggravates the condition. The emotional state of the patient will also be taken into account. All peculiar, rare and significant symptoms, the so-called main or guiding symptoms, will be noted and will help in the search for the remedy that most closely matches the complaint. The remedy will be the substance which would cause similar symptoms if administered in a toxic dose.

Homeopathy is a holistic and highly personalised therapy.

Self-treatment

You can use homeopathic remedies yourself to treat common complaints and minor illnesses successfully.

The Little Book of Homeopathy will show you how. Further reading (see page 125) will deepen your understanding and increase your success rate. Please read carefully the pages on homeopathic potencies (page 16) and the right dosage (page 17).

You do not need to worry about taking the wrong remedy – it will do no harm. But always be aware of the limitations of self-treatment. If the condition is serious, if it does not improve or if you have any concerns, consult a qualified practitioner.

How to find the right remedy

1. Read the brief descriptions of the remedies in Part 2 and choose the remedy that most closely corresponds to your complaint(s), i.e., the most similar one.

2. If you are unsure about which to choose, study the remedies in Part 3 and compare the selected remedies. Once again, choose the remedy that best fits your case.

3. It is always preferable to choose only one remedy; but if necessary you can choose up to three remedies and take them one after the other, at intervals (see page 19).

4. If none of the descriptions matches your symptoms, you cannot help yourself with this book and will need to consult a practitioner.

Homeopathic potencies

Homeopathic remedies are used according to the law of similarities. It is therefore essential that these remedies are administered in a highly diluted form. Only a mild preparation of the substance will give your defence system the information it needs to deal with the illness in the right way without causing any harm to you and your 'life force'.

Samuel Hahnemann developed a method in which the remedy is not only diluted, but also vigorously and rhythmically shaken after each stage of dilution. This has a peculiar effect on the remedy: far from weakening it, as you might expect, this method releases the potency of the substance gradually and makes its healing effects gentler, longer lasting and more powerful. He called this method 'Potenziation'. Consequently, homeopathic remedies are available in different potencies or strengths. The trained homeopath is able to fine-tune his treatment through skilled selection of the appropriate potency.

For use at home the potencies 6c and 30c are the most common and most useful. If the complaint is mainly physical, the potency 6c is used. If there are marked emotional symptoms (irritability, anger, depression, grief, etc.), the potency 30c may prove more effective.

How often should you take a remedy?

The basic rules to remember are:

The right dose
- The more acute the complaint, the more frequently you should take the remedy.

- As soon as your condition improves,

reduce the number of times you take the remedy.

- When you feel well, stop taking the remedy altogether.

For the remedies and potencies listed in this book, you can observe the following:

- **In the potency 6c: take 1 pill 3–6 times a day until your condition improves.**
- **In the potency 30c: take 1 pill 1–3 times a day until your condition improves.**

These recommendations apply to all age groups.

The right way to take the remedy

Put the remedy directly on your tongue (without using a spoon or touching it) and chew it or let it slowly dissolve. For small children the pills can be crushed. Never use metal spoons. To avoid interference with the effect of the remedy, you should not eat, drink or brush your teeth 10 minutes before or after taking it.

If you have difficulty deciding between several remedies, you can select up to a maximum of three. Try one remedy at a time. After an interval of a few hours you can change to your second choice. If neither remedy seems to work, wait another few hours and then take the third remedy.

Certain remedies are recommended in cream or tincture form. In such cases you will find directions in the text on how to use them.

Possible reactions

The remedy works: in this case your condition improves. Initially you often feel a general up-lifting sensation, followed by an improvement in the physical symptoms. As a general rule, acute illnesses respond more quickly to the right remedy and minor, less acute and chronic complaints take longer to respond.

The remedy doesn't work or no longer works: if your condition does not improve or even gradually deteriorates, you have chosen the wrong remedy or possibly the symptoms have changed. Please check the choice of remedy and try to find a more appropriate, more 'similar' one.

Initial aggravation: sometimes, at the beginning of the treatment, a brief flare-up or aggravation of the existing symptoms might appear. This is called an initial aggravation or first reaction. It is initiated by the strengthened self-defence mechanism or immune system and indicates that you have chosen the right remedy. In such cases it is best to stop taking the remedy until this healing reaction has subsided and then resume.

How to store the remedies

Homeopathic remedies should be stored in a dark place, away from strong smelling substances (such as perfumes or essential oils) and kept out of the reach of children.

When should you see a doctor?

The Little Book of Homeopathy recommends self-treatment only for common and minor complaints, for which you would not normally seek immediate help from your GP. Generally speaking you should always see your GP or an experienced homeopath if:

- the symptoms are severe, very acute, unusual or return constantly
- your condition does not improve, or even gets worse
- you feel at all unsure about self-treatment
- conditions have already existed for some time, are chronic, or frequently recur.

The Little Book of Homeopathy cannot take the place of your GP or an experienced homeopathic practitioner!

Side effects and risks?

The remedies in this guide (in their recommended doses and potencies) have no known side effects or negative interactions with any other medication.

However, if you are pregnant or are treating a baby, you should first consult your GP or homeopathic practitioner.

Never stop taking any medication prescribed by your GP, without his or her consent.

There is only one risk with homeopathic self-treatment: this comes not from the remedies themselves but the delay which can occur before the right remedy is identified and taken. If your condition does not improve, see your practitioner sooner rather than later.

The homeopathic kit

For effective self-treatment it is advisable to keep a few remedies at home or with you when travelling. If you have a selection of remedies within easy reach, you can catch common complaints and minor illnesses in their early stages and thereby increase your chances of getting better quickly. All the remedies listed are available from most chemists or health-food shops (see page 123).

Although 44 homeopathic remedies are listed in this book, aproximately 20 remedies should be sufficient to treat most of the complaints listed. You can add to the kit as you become more confident and experienced.

An average basic homeopathic kit should contain the following remedies:

- *Aconite* – colds, fever, cough
- *Apis* – stings, cystitis
- *Arnica* – injuries, bruises
- *Arsenicum album* – diarrhoea, vomiting, food-poisoning
- *Belladonna* – fever, headaches, earaches, inflammations
- *Bryonia* – fever, dry cough, joint ache
- *Cantharis* – cystitis, burns, sunburn
- *Chamomilla* – stomach pain, diarrhoea, teething
- *Gelsemium* – flu, fears
- *Hepar sulphuris* – sore throat, pus, spots
- *Hypericum* – injuries to nerve-endings
- *Ignatia* – grief and sorrow
- *Ledum* – stings, bites, injuries
- *Kali bich* – sinus problems and colds
- *Magnesium phos* – cramps, pain, sciatica

- *Mercurius* – suppuration, sore throat
- *Nux vomica* – nausea, hangover, stress
- *Pulsatilla* – colds, cough, ear and eye infections
- *Rhus toxidendron* – strains and sprains
- *Ruta* – injuries to tendons and ligaments

Additional remedies
- Rescue remedy (drops and cream) – injuries, emergencies
- Arnica (cream) – bruises: apply only if the skin has not been punctured
- Calendula (cream) – sores and infected skin

Apply creams 2–3 times daily or whenever needed.

PART 2

COMPLAINTS FROM A TO Z

In this chapter you will find common complaints and illnesses listed in alphabetical order. To find the right remedy for your condition look under the appropriate heading(s) and compare the description of each remedy with the symptoms of your complaint. Choose the remedy associated with the symptoms that most closely correspond to your condition. If more than one remedy seems suitable and you are unsure which one to select, you should refer to the remedy 'profiles' in Part 3.

For guidance on how to take the remedies refer to Part 1.

ABSCESS
See page 31.

ANXIETY
See page 46.

BITES
See page 64.

BLADDER COMPLAINTS and CYSTITIS

- If you feel the constant urge to pass water, even after you have just been to the toilet or you keep making visits to the toilet for fear of not being able to hold back the urine, try *Apis* – an effective remedy for cystitis. You may also suffer from burning or severe stinging pains.

- If you experience a burning pain when you urinate and a constant, overwhelming urge to pass water, but find that you can only pass a few drops, try *Cantharis*, the main homeopathic remedy for cystitis. If the cystitis is more severe, there are often sharp pains before, during and after urination.

- For acute inflammation with cramping and burning pains, aggravated by the slightest jolt or pressure and, in some cases, accompanied by high fever, take *Belladonna*.

- In both of the following cases, warmth alleviates the condition. If you suffer from an irritable bladder after catching cold, getting wet or being physically overworked, and your whole body aches, *Rhus tox* can be very effective. Alternatively, if you are spending a lot of stressful time sitting behind a desk, you will need *Nux vomica*.

- Repeated bouts of cystitis often brought

on by catching cold and getting wet feet can result in an irritable bladder with frequent incontinence (especially when coughing or laughing). In this case try *Pulsatilla*.

- For cramp-like symptoms that make you double up in pain and leave you feeling irritable and angry, *Colocynthis* will bring relief.

BLOATEDNESS, DISTENSION and WIND

- *Carbo veg* can help in cases where the upper part of the stomach feels bloated, the abdomen is tight and tense, you are burping and producing foul wind, and you long for fresh air.
- *Lycopodium* might be the right remedy when the lower abdomen is bloated, there is inoffensive wind and loud rumbling noises, and you cannot bear anything tight

around your stomach. The symptoms are worse in the afternoon and early evening.

- Bloatedness, constipation and cramping pains (especially after indulgence and/or too much alcohol) are symptoms that often respond well to *Nux vomica*.

- If you feel bloated after eating sugar and sweets and your stomach is very distended, *Arg nit* might help, especially if you are a nervous or fearful person.

BOILS, ABCESSES and SUPPURATION

- For the initial inflammation and to avoid subsequent suppuration, *Arnica* is extremely effective. If the area becomes red, hot, swollen and throbbing, take *Belladonna*.

- If pus then forms, the area is extremely sensitive to touch, and the pain is sharp and stinging, *Hepar sulph* is the best remedy. If taken early enough, it can prevent the formation of pus.

- If a boil develops very slowly, *Silica* will accelerate the healing process, especially if you suffer from spots and acne which have a tendency to develop slowly. The remedy usually causes the pus to form more quickly and helps the abscess to open. It also helps to ease splinters out from under the skin.

BONES, injured or broken

- As with all other injuries, *Arnica* should be taken in the first instance.
- For injured joints or concussion of a bone (e.g., of the shin), *Ruta* will often help.
- If you have to keep completely still because every movement is extremely painful, *Bryonia* is likely to be the right remedy.
- If a bone is broken or partly broken, *Symphytum* will speed up the healing process and might ease the pain a little.

The bone should of course first be set by a doctor.

BRUISES
See page 52.

BURNS, SCALDS and SUNBURN

- For the initial shock caused by the injury, *Arnica* and *Rescue remedy* can always be taken.

- For minor burns and scalding, *Rescue* cream or drops work extremely well. If used quickly (apply the drops if the cream is not available), the remedy can even prevent the formation of blisters.

- If the skin is red, hot, perhaps even slightly swollen (common signs of sunburn) and you also feel a throbbing pain, you should try *Belladonna*.

- If you suffer from severe burning pains and

your skin develops blisters, *Cantharis* will often bring relief.

COLDS and RUNNY NOSE
See page 61.

COLDS and FLU
- For colds which start suddenly, often at night, which are perhaps caused by a cold wind and involve initial chills followed by a high fever with hot dry skin, acute thirst and restlessness, consider taking *Aconite*. If this remedy is taken in the early stages, it can often stop the cold in its tracks.

- If the condition starts suddenly, caused by wet cold weather, and you have a high fever but the skin is hot and moist, your face is red and your head aches, *Belladonna* is preferable.

- If the cold begins with chills, trembling and the chattering of teeth, you feel tired, weak and floppy and suffer from headache, muscle ache and sore throat, take *Gelsemium*, especially for a summer flu and if your face is dark red in colour.

- For flu with intense bone- and muscle-ache or a 'battered and bruised' sensation, *Arnica* and *Rhus tox* are both helpful. If you also suffer from fever and headaches, *Eupatorium* might be preferable.

- For a cold that develops slowly, accompanied by intense thirst, irritability and a strong desire to be left alone in peace to rest, consider *Bryonia*.

- Should you suffer from a burning, watery thin nasal discharge and feel weak and chilly with a desire for warmth and warm drinks, *Arsenicum* will be best.

CONJUNCTIVITIS
See page 44.

CONSTIPATION

- For constipation with a dry, hard stool and a strong desire for cold drinks, consider *Bryonia*.

- For constipation caused by stress, by an abuse of laxatives or when routine is upset, take *Nux vomica*. You often feel a cramp-like urge to pass a stool, but are unable to do so.

- If you pass a dry, hard stool only after a great deal of effort and you feel the stool slipping back despite all the pushing and pressing, try *Silica*.

- If you feel constipated and bloated and the stool is initially hard but then becomes soft and is passed in large amounts, *Lycopodium* is probably the right remedy. You may also find it difficult to pass stools on unfamiliar toilets.

COUGH

- For a sudden cough that appears mainly at night, with dry, violent attacks and possibly with wheezing, *Aconite* is recommended.

- If the cough develops slowly, is dry and sounds hard, and you perhaps find yourself clutching your chest when you cough to avoid the pain, take *Byronia*, a very helpful remedy for the common dry cough. You usually feel very thirsty (for cold drinks).

- For a spastic, irritating cough with frequent coughing attacks that take your breath away and might even lead to retching or vomiting, try *Drosera*.

- If you have a suffocating, dry, barking, spasmodic, sawing cough and your voice is throaty, try *Spongia*.

- A painful, barking cough that brings up gluey yellow-green phlegm, and an extreme aversion to cold will often improve with *Hepar sulph*.

- If you suffer from a rattling in the chest with a sticky phlegm which is difficult to cough up, and retching, vomiting and nausea, try the remedy *Ipecac*.
- For those (small children or old people in particular) who suffer from a rattling cough, with a glutinous whitish phlegm which is difficult to cough up and leaves you feeling exhausted and out of breath, consider *Ant tart*.
- A loose cough with yellowish or green phlegm which gets coughed up easily in the mornings, will often react well to *Pulsatilla*.
- For a dry cough, which does not subside after taking *Bryonia*, accompanied by chest pain, intense thirst or marked hoarseness, consider *Phosphorus*.

CUTS

See page 71.

CYSTITIS
See page 28.

DENTIST / OPERATIONS,
before and after

- If you feel anxious or fearful about an operation or a visit to the dentist, take *Gelsemium*, *Arg nit* or *Rescue remedy*.

- For any injury, including dental treatment or surgical operations, *Arnica* is extremely effective. One dose before the treatment or operation, followed by the normal dosage, three times a day, will enhance the healing process. Externally, apply *Calendula* cream or *Hypericum* cream to the skin.

- Bleeding (e.g., after the extraction of a tooth) can often be stopped by taking the remedy *Phosphorus*.

- For clear cuts or puncture wounds, such as those caused by endoscopy, episiotomy, biopsy or catheter, try *Staphysagria*.

- If a nerve is injured, you may feel shooting pains along the nerve. In such cases, try *Hypericum*.

- If you have problems regaining complete consciousness after an anaesthetic, you could consider *Phosphorus*. For persistent nausea *Nux vomica* and *Ipecac* will often help.

DIGESTIVE PROBLEMS: DIARRHOEA, NAUSEA and VOMITING

- *Nux vomica* is the most important remedy for nausea with ineffective retching. Your food feels like a stone in your stomach, and you may be angry and irritable.

- For cases of slight food poisoning with diarrhoea, vomiting, weakness, restlessness, anxiety and a feeling of being constantly cold, *Arsenicum* is an extremely useful remedy.

- If the vomiting and diarrhoea are accompanied by cold sweats and weakness, as if you are close to fainting, and the slightest movement sets off the need to vomit or to pass stools, you should try *Veratrum*.

- If your stomach is extremely bloated, you have to belch constantly, you feel short of breath and long for fresh air although you feel cold, consider *Carbo veg*.

- If you suffer from nausea or possibly the vomiting of bile, especially after eating too much fat or fatty greasy food, pork or ice-cream, then *Pulsatilla* or *Carbo veg* are recommended. The symptoms improve after gentle exercise and fresh air. Stuffy, airless rooms are unbearable.

- For constant nausea and retching not relieved by vomiting, *Ipecac* can be very effective.

DISTENSION and WIND

See page 30.

EAR COMPLAINTS

- In the early stages of a middle ear infection with a slow onset, *Ferrum phos* is the most important remedy. You should take it as soon as possible.

- If you awake suddenly at night with unbearable earache, or if the pains are caused by a cold wind, take *Aconite* immediately.

- For a sudden, intense and throbbing earache with a red, hot face and possibly high fever, try *Belladonna*. This is the main remedy for acute middle-ear infections.

- If you suffer from an unbearable, stinging earache, that makes you extremely irritable, consider *Chamomilla*. The patient (usually a child), cries angrily, throws itself from side to side, and often wants to be carried. One cheek may be red, the other pale.

- If, on the other hand, the patient is quiet, weepy, very dependent and clingy, and even wants to be in the fresh air, *Pulsatilla* is preferable. Sometimes you will find a mild, yellow-green discharge coming out of the ear.

- Earache caused by cold air or a draft, which is worse when you swallow and better when you are warm, often improves with *Nux vomica*. You may feel irritable and stressed, and sometimes even the hair on your scalp may be sensitive to the touch.

- For cases of stinging earache, in which the slightest cold makes the pain worse, and you feel compelled to cover up the ear to keep it warm, consider *Hepar sulph*. Sometimes there will be a yellow-green discharge coming out of the ear. The patient is extremely irritable.

- If you have discharge from the ear, swollen lymph-nodes under the ear, bad breath, night sweats and thirst, *Mercurius* can alleviate your symptoms.

EYE INFLAMMATION and CONJUCTIVITIS

- *Euphrasia*, eyebright, is commonly used for all burning pains in the eye, when the eye feels as if there is sand in it, causing it to water and be sensitive to bright light. Dissolve some eyebright granules in clean, boiled water and use this to wash the eye carefully. It is possible to do this with a tea made from the eyebright herb, too.

- If the eyes are dry, hot and feel gritty (as if you had sand in them), you may need *Aconite*. This remedy is effective in cases where the symptoms are very acute and sudden, often triggered by a cold wind, eye strain or foreign bodies in the eye.

- Bright red eyes, extreme sensitivity to light and throbbing pains often respond well to *Belladonna*.

- If the eyelids are heavily swollen, there are stinging pains, and cold applications bring relief, consider *Apis*.

- If there are profuse mild, yellowish and viscous tears which coagulate the eyelids, *Pulsatilla* is often helpful.

EYE INJURIES

- For any injury to the eyes, *Arnica*, the main remedy for injuries in general, should be taken in the first instance.

- In cases where the pain is very acute and sudden, e.g., caused by a foreign body, take *Aconite*.

- If the eye is irritated, *Euphrasia* can also be taken.

- For a black eye (e.g., from a blow),

Symphytum alternated with *Ledum* often works well.

- If the eye is swollen following an injury and the swelling is not hot (but cold applications bring relief), it is best to take *Ledum*.

EYE STRAIN

- For eye strain caused by reading, bad light and extensive work in front of a computer screen, *Ruta* alternated with *Euphrasia* is the best remedy.

FEARS, ANXIETY and PANIC

- For a sudden feeling of panic, intense fear of dying, shock and terror (e.g., after an accident), for acute claustrophobia or for anxiety during acute illness, consider *Aconite* and *Rescue* drops.

- For a fear of forthcoming events, such as a journey or an interview, try *Arg nit*. You constantly feel in a hurry, are possibly claustrophobic, may have a fear of flying or of heights and a craving for sweet things.

- If you have a nervous fear of exams or interviews, or suffer from stage fright, with trembling, weakness, loose stools and a feeling of failure, *Gelsemium* can work wonders.

- People who suffer from the cold, from a feeling of great anxiety and panic, who feel very weak and internally restless, may respond well to *Arsenicum*. The condition is aggravated by loneliness and darkness.

FEVER

- In cases of rapidly rising, very high temperatures, *Aconite* and *Belladonna* should first be considered. If there is also thirst, dry hot skin, no sweating, restlessness and anxiety, *Aconite* is the better remedy.

- If your skin is hot, moist and damp, your face is red, your hand and feet cold and you have throbbing pains and feel dazed, *Belladonna* is the better choice.
- For a slow-developing, middle-high fever without any other significant symptoms, *Ferrum phos.* should be given. It works especially well in the early stages of an infection.
- Consider the flu remedy *Gelsemium* if you have fever, tiredness, weakness, chills, shivering and possibly a dark red face.
- If the whole body feels hot, and the face is red and hot, but throwing off the covers makes you shiver, then *Nux vomica* is a good choice.
- For fever with an intense thirst, irritability and a desire to be left in absolute peace, *Bryonia* should be considered.
- Weepy and clingy children, who do not

want to be on their own and need physical comfort when they feel unwell, respond best to *Pulsatilla*.

FLU
See page 34.

GRIEF and WORRIES
- *Ignatia* can ease some of the grief caused by the loss of a loved one, love sickness or even homesickness – especially if you sigh a lot, feel oversensitive, suffer from mood swings and are perhaps even a bit hysterical.
- If you cry constantly and want to be comforted, taken care of and surrounded by loved ones, *Pulsatilla* is preferable.
- For the acute shock caused by the loss of a loved one, *Rescue remedy* is often extremely helpful.

HANGOVER

- For headaches, nausea, retching, heartburn or spasmodic stomach ache after too much alcohol, smoking or over-indulgence, *Nux vomica* is the first and most important remedy. If you take it at night with plenty of water, the worst effects can often be avoided.

HAYFEVER

- For constant sneezing and watery acrid nasal discharge, but no acrid watering eyes, *Allium cepa* is a very helpful remedy, especially if the symptoms seem to get worse in a warm environment.

- Constant sneezing and a sharp burning sensation, coupled with a thin, watery nasal discharge which gets worse in the cold, will respond better to *Arsenicum*. This remedy also works for noses that are more blocked at night and asthmatic wheezing.

- If the eyes are red and watering, and you shed acrid tears, which make the corners of the eyes sore, try *Euphrasia*. (The eyes are inflamed and very sensitive to light, you sneeze a lot and your nose runs with a mild discharge.)
- Nelson's homeopathic *Hayfever tablets* are of great value in many cases of hayfever.

HOARSENESS
- Sudden hoarseness resulting from an acute cold (caused by a cold wind) responds well to *Aconite*.
- If there is loss of voice mainly in the evening or after too much talking or singing, try *Phosphorus*.
- For hoarseness which is worse in the mornings and after breaks from talking, and which improves with talking, you should take *Rhus tox*.
- For hoarseness accompanied by a barking

cough (laryngitis) *Drosera*, *Spongia* or *Hepar sulph* are reliable remedies.

INJURY and BRUISES

- In any accident or injury the first remedy you should consider is *Arnica*. As the most effective homeopathic remedy for any kind of injury, Arnica helps with bruising and bleeding and enhances the healing process. It is also a wonderful remedy for the shock caused by injuries. Take the remedy at short intervals until you feel better. In addition to the tablets, you can apply Arnica cream to bruises, but only if the skin is unbroken.

- *Rescue remedy* helps to ease shock and panic of any kind. You can take the drops on their own or in combination with *Arnica*. Apply 3–4 drops on the tongue or lips, if necessary at short intervals. *Rescue* cream can be applied to the injured area on its own or alternated with the *Arnica* cream.

- Injuries of the nerves or of tissues which are rich in nerves, will often create shooting, pulling pains along the nerve. In such cases *Hypericum* will often help. Crushed fingers and toes, concussion of the coccyx, scratches and sores on the palms, or injuries to the lips, inner mouth or ear, respond very well to this remedy.

INSOMNIA
See page 62.

JET LAG
See page 70.

LUMBAGO and SCIATICA

- If you have sudden, severe pain aggravated by the slightest movement and an intolerance to warm applications, take *Aconite*, the remedy for acute conditions.
- When you ache and feel bruised, sore and

limping, as if someone has beaten you up, and even the bed feels too hard, try *Arnica*. The condition improves with rest and warmth.

- If initial movements feel stiff, painful and strained but improve with gentle, continuous movement, then *Rhus tox* may be your remedy. In such cases warmth will always help.

- If, on the contrary, you have to keep absolutely still because the slightest movement causes unbearable pain, *Bryonia* is the more appropriate remedy.

- *Nux vomica* should be considered if the pain is worse when you move and better in the warmth, and you have to sit up to be able to turn around in bed.

- For sciatica, with neuralgic pains shooting down the leg, *Mag phos* and *Colocynthis* are both effective remedies.

MENOPAUSE

- If you experience frequent hot flushes alternating with chills, cannot bear anything tight around your throat, and feel worse after sleep, consider *Lachesis*. You often have the strong desire to talk a lot and rapidly, and you may feel easily jealous and irritable.

- *Sepia* is a helpful remedy in cases where the slightest exertion makes you sweat, you feel completely exhausted, washed out, and overburdened by your job, your partner and your family, and you wish you could leave it all behind. In women a bearing down sensation in the uterus often makes you cross your legs, when sitting.

- If you are weepy, moody, longing for company and sympathy, you suffer from hot flushes and have a desire for fresh air, try *Pulsatilla*. At night, after you have fallen asleep, you often start to sweat profusely.

MUSCLE ACHE, SPRAINS and STRAINS

- For muscle ache or pulled muscles with a 'beaten-up' sensation, *Arnica* is a very reliable remedy. To avoid muscle ache, one dose of the remedy can be given as a preventative.

- If not just the muscles themselves, but also the tendons, ligaments and joints are strained or sprained or bones are bruised, *Arnica* will not be sufficient on its own. In such cases you should also take *Ruta*.

- For sprains and strains that are initially painful when you move, but which then improve with gentle, continuous movement, *Rhus tox* will often bring rapid relief.

- If you have to keep the injured area completely still, because even the slightest movement is unbearably painful, then you

need *Bryonia*. Tight pressure or
bandages may often alleviate the pain.

NAUSEA
See page 40.

NOSE BLEEDS
- If the nose bleed has been caused by an
  injury or blow, you should first take *Arnica*.
- If the blood is bright red, try *Ferrum phos*.
- For frequent bleeding with a lot of bright
  red blood, *Phosphorus* can bring good
  results.

OPERATIONS, before and after
See page 39.

PANIC
See page 46.

PERIOD PAIN

- If the pain makes you bend double and the symptoms respond well to warmth or gentle pressure or massage of the stomach, you should try *Mag phos*. The pain stops with the onset of the bleeding.

- If the pain makes you bend double, comes and goes in waves and you feel angry and irritable, you should consider *Colocynthis*. In such cases you often press your fist against your stomach, because tight pressure seems to alleviate the pain. The pain starts with the onset of the period.

- Unbearable pain with hot flushes and sweating often responds well to *Chamomilla*. You are beside yourself with pain. You often snap at other people and feel extremely irritable.

- Other remedies, such as *Pulsatilla*, *Sepia*, *Lachesis* and *Nux vomica*, listed under pre-menstrual tension below can also be helpful, if their emotional symptoms correspond closely to your condition.

PREMENSTRUAL TENSION (PMT)

- If you feel very moody and exceptionally weepy, long for company, sympathy and consolation and cannot bear to be alone, the most likely remedy is *Pulsatilla*. You often have a desire for fresh air. Sticky, warm rooms are intolerable. Your breasts are usually swollen and painful before your period.

- If, on the contrary, you feel irritable and as if you would like to leave your job, your partner or family, or you feel sad, despondent and depressed, consider *Sepia*. You may be completely exhausted, but feel better after vigorous exercise.

- Try *Lachesis* if you feel exceptionally talkative, irritable, quarrelsome and envious. All symptoms improve with the onset of your period. You cannot bear anything tight around your throat or stomach and you feel much worse in a warm environment or after sleep.

- Women who are irritable, angry and sensitive to the cold (cold winds and drafts), irritated by noise and smells, and who have a hectic, stressful lifestyle, often combined with an abuse of alcohol, medication and drugs, should consider *Nux vomica*.

PUNCTURE WOUNDS

- For puncture wounds caused by, for example, thorns, needles, splinters, nails, etc., take *Arnica* tablets as the first remedy.

- After *Arnica*, the most important homeopathic remedy is *Ledum*, especially if the area that has been punctured starts to swell, is dark in colour and feels cold, but is alleviated by cold applications.

- If there are pulling or shooting pains along the nerves, try *Hypericum*.

RUNNY NOSE

- To treat a runny nose with lots of sneezing, a watery acrid discharge and a desire for warmth and warm drinks, try *Arsenicum*.

- Take *Allium cepa* for a cold with a lot of sneezing, a watery, burning discharge, weeping eyes and a desire for fresh air.

- If you catch colds easily from getting cold or from a draft, if there is a thin watery, clear discharge and lots of sneezing, if the nose runs during the day but feels bunged up in the evenings and in a warm environment, *Nux vomica* is recommended.

- For thick, ropy, stringy, yellow-green mucus, or glutinous bogies obstructing the nose, *Kali bich* is a wonderful remedy.

- A lot of mild, thick, yellow-green mucus in the mornings and a blocked nose at night are symptoms that respond well to *Pulsatilla*.

SCALDS
See page 33.

SCIATICA
See page 54.

SLEEP, disturbed and INSOMNIA
- If you wake up feeling anxious, with a wild, pounding heart or the acute fear of imminent death, *Aconite* will bring you some peace of mind. This remedy is also helpful for treating insomnia caused by

internal restlessness, emotional upsets, anger or fear.

- If you have a fear and apprehension of coming events, consider *Arg nit*.

- If you feel nervous, as if you have drunk too much coffee, and your mind is racing so much you cannot get to sleep, *Coffea* (homeopathically prepared coffee) will calm you down.

- If you have to work night shifts or suffer from the effects of intercontinental air travel (jet lag), a disturbed sleep pattern or lack of sleep, and you are dizzy with exhaustion but still cannot sleep, *Cocculus* is the best remedy.

- Workaholics and stressed 'city people' with an over-excited nervous system, who wake up too early and in a filthy mood often need *Nux vomica*. It is also recommended after over-indulgence and an excess of coffee, nicotine, alcohol or drugs.

- If you feel battered and bruised and, worn out after physical exertion, and even the bed seems too hard, *Arnica* may help you to sleep.

SORE THROAT

- When a sore throat suddenly flares up (often triggered by dry, cold weather) and you feel extremely thirsty for cold water, try *Aconite*. It is most effective if taken in the early stages of illness.

- If your throat is dry and bright red, with burning or even throbbing pains, and you have to swallow constantly even though it hurts to do so, *Belladonna* is the best remedy.

- For stinging pains and pink-red, glossy, shining, swollen tonsils, throat and uvula, soothed by cold drinks, *Apis* is recommended.

- If the throat is dark red, the glands of the neck and lower jaw are swollen, and the pain extends to the ear when you swallow, consider *Phytolacca*.

- If the sore throat is worse on the left side and the throat is dark red or purple and if the swallowing, especially of hot drinks, is very painful and you cannot bear anything tight around the neck, try *Lachesis*.

- When the sore throat is caused by cold or a draught, and the throat is red, swallowing is painful, the pain extends to the ear, and you feel irritable and angry, *Nux vomica* often helps. Warm drinks also help.

- For sharp stinging pains, as though you had a fish bone stuck in your throat, extreme pain each time you swallow, and acute aversion to the cold, consider *Hepar sulph*.

SORES

See page 71.

SPRAIN and STRAINS

see page 56.

STINGS and BITES

- For symptoms that resemble a bee sting that swells and is pale-red, with a stinging pain that is soothed by cold applications, try *Apis*.

- If the swelling is of a darker colour and the area feels cold but cold applications seem to help, *Ledum* is preferable. This is the most important remedy for mosquito, tick and animal bites.

- For stings and bites in tissues that are rich in nerves (lips, tongue, ears, palms, etc.), and for shooting neuralgic pain, take *Hypericum*.

- If the area is bruised, consider *Arnica*.

- For minor stings and bites the *Rescue* or *Calendula* cream may be all you need.

STOMACH ACHE

- Colic-like stomach ache that makes you double up in pain usually responds well to *Colocynthis*.

- For colic-like stomach ache that improves with warm applications (e.g., hot water bottle) and tender massaging of the stomach, try *Mag phos*.

- Colic-like stomach pains that come and go suddenly and which may force you to bend double or backwards in order to ease them, respond well to *Belladonna*. The stomach is very sensitive to pressure and touch, and you may feel hot and sweaty.

- For cramp-like stomach ache, often accompanied by wind, bloatedness and constipation, that flares up a few hours after eating, consider *Nux vomica*. You feel easily irritable, angry and stressed.

STYES

- The most common remedy is *Staphysagria*. It is even beneficial for recurring styes. Women and children should also consider *Pulsatilla*.

SUNBURN

See page 33.

TOOTHACHE

- For sudden, severe toothache, especially if triggered by cold, *Aconite* can bring fast relief.
- If there is more of a throbbing pain and if the area is red and inflamed, take *Belladonna*.
- Unbearable raging toothache, which makes you irritable, and allows you no rest, often

responds to *Chamomilla*. Warmth makes
the condition worse.

- If you suffer from tooth decay, if cold
  makes the condition worse and if you feel
  extremely irritable and angry, try *Hepar
  sulph*.
- For caries, decay, pain, ulcers, bad breath,
  a metallic taste in the mouth and an
  increased production of saliva, *Mercurius* is
  an effective remedy. Neither hot nor cold
  is tolerated.
- For shooting neuralgic pains in the region
  of the jaw and teeth, *Mag phos* is
  recommended.

TRAVELLER'S NERVES
- If you feel apprehensive and frantic several
  days before departure, *Arg nit* will calm you
  down. It is, incidentally, also a very useful
  remedy for claustrophobia.

- If you are shaking with fear before departure, and you feel weak and tired, *Gelsemium* will give you strength.
- For sudden panic attacks, fears and frights, *Aconite* and *Rescue remedy*, given in frequent doses before and during the journey, can be very effective.

TRAVEL SICKNESS and JET LAG
- Some people (and many children) suffer from nausea, vomiting and vertigo when travelling in a boat, car or plane. *Cocculus* may alleviate the symptoms. This remedy also works well in cases of Jet lag.

VOMITING
See page 40.

WORRIES
See page 46.

WOUNDS: SORES and CUTS

- The first remedies you should consider are *Arnica* and/or *Hypericum*.

- To enhance the healing process, you can apply *Calendula* or *Hypericum* cream. Apply the cream 2–3 times daily. *Tip*: For mouth ulcers, apply a few drops of *Hypericum tincture*. It stings for a moment but works wonders.

- For clean cuts use *Staphysagria,* and for punctured wounds take *Ledum*.

Homeopathy for children and babies

Children often respond extremely well to homeopathic remedies. However, given that it is not always possible to ask children many questions, you have to rely more upon close, accurate observation. This can make it harder to select the right remedy. Generally speaking, all the recommendations in *The Little Book of Homeopathy* also apply to the treatment of children, but in this chapter you will find some advice specific to children and babies.

In the case of any serious illness, you should consult your GP, but common complaints can often be treated quickly, gently and effectively with homeopathic remedies. Nevertheless, always be aware of the limitations of self-treatment (see page 22).

COLIC

- Spastic stomach ache, which improves with warmth, gentle massage and rubbing of the stomach, often responds well to *Mag phos*.

- If the child draws his legs up to his stomach, cries out angrily, and is quite irritable, *Colocynthis* may be preferable. Warmth, pressure (lying on the stomach) and the passing of wind bring relief.

- If the belly is bloated like a drum, the child is extremely irritable and constantly crying, his head is red, hot and sweaty, and the only thing that seems to help is to carry him around, try *Chamomilla*.

- Among sensitive children spastic stomach aches may develop after grief, punishment and a feeling of being unloved, and will often respond well to *Ignatia*.

CROUP (cough) (see also page 37)
- For a dry, barking croup-like cough,

Aconite, Drosera, Spongia and *Hepar sulph.* can produce very good results. Study the remedies and choose the one best suited to your child's condition. If you are still unsure which to choose, you can try each of the remedies in the above order until you find the right one.

DIARRHOEA (see also page 40)

- For spastic pain and greenish diarrhoea that looks like chopped spinach and may smell of rotten eggs, try *Chamomilla*. The child is extremely irritable, hurls himself from side to side and wants to be carried.

DIGESTIVE PROBLEMS
(see also page 40)

- Spastic stomach ache after too much or too rich food (e.g., after a birthday party), with nausea and retching, will often improve with *Nux vomica*.

- If the nausea and digestive problems are

caused by greasy food, pastry, pork or ice-cream and the child seems to feel better when moving gently in the fresh air, *Pulsatilla* may be the best remedy.

FEVER (see also page 48)
- At the onset of every feverish condition *Ferrum phos* should be considered, especially for slow-developing fever up to 39°C (102°F), with a pale-red, blotched face and occasional bleeding from the nose.
- Sudden high fevers above 39°C (102°F) often respond well to *Aconite* or *Belladonna* (and *Eupatorium*). A high fever normally indicates a healthy and fast-reacting immune system, but if you feel at all unsure, consult your GP or homeopath.

TEETHING
- Consider *Mag phos* if rubbing, chewing, biting (e.g., on a dummy) and warmth seem to bring relief.

- If the child is extremely irritable and moody, if one cheek is red and the other pale, and nothing seems to calm him down except being carried around, *Chamomilla* will often help.

- If on the contrary the child is quiet, very weepy and moody, does not want to be left alone and needs comfort and sympathy, *Pulsatilla* will be the better remedy. *Chamomilla* and *Pulsatilla* apply to cases where there is an aversion to warmth.

PART 3

THE REMEDIES FROM A–Z

In this chapter you will find a brief introduction to each of the 44 homeopathic remedies mentioned in *The Little Book of Homeopathy*. Under each remedy you will find some of the complaints and symptoms known to respond well to that remedy. This is followed by a list of the main associated symptoms.

This information should help confirm your choice of remedy, especially if you have difficulty deciding between several. For guidance on how to use the remedies, refer to Part 1.

Aconite

Monkshood – *Aconite napallus*

First recommendation for treating colds in their early stages.

Recommended:

For all acute or feverish complaints that appear suddenly and with intensity. For best results, take the remedy as soon as the symptoms appear.

Main symptoms:

- often caused by dry cold, cold wind, panic and shock
- complaints come suddenly and are extremely fierce
- fever rises rapidly and may be very high, with a hot, dry skin
- patient is extremely restless and anxious
- intense thirst for cold drinks

Allium cepa

Onion – *Allium cepa*

Recommended:

For hayfever and colds, if the following symptoms arise:

Main symptoms:

- often caused by cold, wet and damp conditions
- constant sneezing and a runny nose
- nose and eyes are red and irritated
- acrid, watery nasal discharge which makes the nostrils sore, but mild tears
- itching and scraping in the throat
- you feel worse in the evenings and in the warmth; better in cool conditions

Ant tart

Tartar emetic – *Antimonium tartaricum*

Recommended:

For coughs and bronchitis with lots of phlegm, especially in young children and the elderly. It helps to bring up mucus.

Main symptoms:

- rattling in the chest with a moist cough; phlegm is coughed up only with difficulty
- moist cough with shortness of breath and wheezing
- cough with vomiting or retching of phlegm
- desire for warmth, but warmth is not tolerated
- weak and pale appearance
- better when sitting up or coughing up phlegm

Apis

Bee – *Apis mellifica*
First recommendation for stings and bites.

Recommended:
For stings and bites, especially bee stings; for sore throats and cystitis, and all conditions which resemble the symptoms of a bee sting.

Main symptoms:
• burning and stinging pain
• pale red, hot swelling
• the painful area is very sensitive
• throat or bladder feel constricted
• no thirst
• you feel worse in the warmth, and better after a cold bath, or cold applications

Arg nit

Silver nitrate – *Argentum nitricum*
First recommendation for anticipatory fears.

Recommended:
For nervousness, panic, anxiety and certain fears; for vertigo, diarrhoea and bloatedness.

Main symptoms:
- panic and fears: claustrophobia, a fear of heights, flying, illness or hospitals
- anxiety and fear of imminent events, e.g., an interview, an exam, a journey, etc.
- you feel in a constant hurry and are worried you will arrive late
- this nervous state may cause diarrhoea
- you may have a strong desire for sweets, often followed by bloatedness and wind

Arnica

Mountain daisy – *Arnica montana*
Highly recommended as a first aid remedy.

Recommended:
For all kinds of injuries, muscle ache, bleeding, flu and sleeplessness.

Main symptoms:
- shock following an injury
- bruises, contusion, strains
- muscle ache and physical exertion
- you feel sore and lame, 'battered and bruised'
- you may feel oversensitive and not want to be touched; even the bed may feel too hard

Arsenicum

Arsenic trioxide – *Arsenicum album*
First recommendation for slight food poisoning.

Recommended:
For food poisoning with vomiting and diarrhoea, colds and asthmatic coughs, insomnia.

Main symptoms:
- you feel cold, weak, restless and anxious
- the slightest exertion is utterly exhausting
- diarrhoea, vomiting and spastic stomach cramps
- cold with a runny nose, cough with wheezing
- burning pains
- desire for warmth and warm drinks
- symptoms are worse at night, in damp and cold conditions and when left alone

Belladonna

Deadly nightshade – *Atropa Belladonna*
*First recommendation for acute throbbing
inflammations and high fevers.*

Recommended:
For acute inflammations, cramping and
throbbing complaints and high fever.

Main symptoms:
- often brought on by cold wet weather or
  wet hair
- the symptoms start suddenly (often
  disappearing as suddenly as they came)
- high fever, red face, little thirst, moist,
  sweaty skin, a desire not to be uncovered
- when feverish you feel either drowsy or
  irritable but not anxious (as with Aconite)
- throbbing, burning, cramping pain with red,
  hot, inflamed areas (e.g., throat, ear)
- sensitivity to movement, light and noise

Bryonia

White bryony – *Bryonia alba*

First recommendation for dry painful coughs.

Recommended:

For dry coughs, constipation, aching joints and backache.

Main symptoms:

- often caused by anger and (financial) worries
- the slightest movement is intolerable, only total rest helps
- you feel irritable and long for peace and quiet
- very thirsty for lots of cold drinks
- stitching pains
- dry cough, which is painful in the chest and hurts the head
- eased by pressure (e.g., holding chest, bandaging joints) and by rest

Calendula

Marigold – *Calendula officinalis*
First recommendation for wounds, sores and cuts.

Recommended:
Calendula enhances and speeds up the healing process and, thanks to its antiseptic properties, can prevent infection and suppuration. Apply as a cream 2–3 times daily or when needed. For the best results, combine with Arnica (apply Calendula as a cream and take Arnica as granules or tablets).

Main symptoms:
• sores, cuts, burns and wounds
• red inflamed wounds with stinging pains
• sore feet or blisters on feet (from walking in uncomfortable shoes)

Cantharis

Spanish fly – *Lytta vesicatoria*
First recommendation for bladder infections.

Recommended:
For cystitis, burns, scalds and sunburn.

Main symptoms:
- severe raw, burning pains
- burning, cutting pains before, during and after passing water
- urine can only be passed drop by drop and burns like fire
- constant urge to pass water
- burning or even blistering of the skin or the internal linings
- sexual organs may be painful and hypersensitive

Carbo veg

Charcoal – *Carbo vegetabilis*

Recommended:
For bloatedness, digestive problems, fainting and collapse.

Main symptoms:
- intense distension of the stomach with shortness of breath and burping
- intolerance to rich or fatty foods and alcohol
- nausea, dizziness and ringing in the ears
- strong desire for air, preferably fanned air
- the body is cold (although the head may be hot)
- severe weakness and a tendency to collapse, with a bluish face or lips (lack of oxygen)

Chamomilla

Camomile – *Matricaria Chamomilla*

First recommendation for teething children.

Recommended:

For teething children, diarrhoea, colic and earache.

Main symptoms:

- unbearable pain
- very irritable, moody and easily enraged; nothing seems to satisfy them
- children want to be carried
- one cheek may be red, the other pale
- often hot, restless and thirsty
- colic pains and possibly greenish diarrhoea that looks like chopped spinach and smells of rotten eggs

Cocculus

Indian cockle – *Anamirta Cocculus*

First recommendation for travel sickness.

Recommended:

For travel sickness, vertigo, disturbed sleep and jet lag.

Main symptoms:

- ill effects of lack of sleep, night shifts, exertion, worry or grief
- an unbalanced walk, from dizziness and weakness
- vertigo with nausea and vomiting, worse when you move and when you get up from bed; better when you lie or sit still
- extra sensitivity to noise
- muscular weakness and nervous exhaustion

Coffea

Coffeebean – *Coffea cruda*

Recommended:

For nervousness, insomnia, over-excitement, palpitations.

Main symptoms:

- ill effects of over-excitement, joy, shock, fright and anger
- mental over-activity, possibly preventing sleep
- nervous palpitations
- coffee or tea have adverse effect
- oversensitivity to pain
- very sensitive hearing

Colocynthis

Bitter cucumber – *Citrullus Colocynthis*

First recommendation for spasmodic pain that makes you bend double.

Recommended:
For spasmodic pain, colic, menstrual pain and sciatica.

Main symptoms:
- often caused by anger and resentment; you feel very irritable when ill
- cramps and colic; bent double with pain
- eased by pressure (babies lie on their tummies)
- sciatica with numbness; you have to bend your leg to relieve the pain
- you feel better after resting, drinking coffee and in a warm environment (e.g., in bed)

Drosera

Sundew – *Drosera rotundifolia*

Recommended:
For dry, spasmodic coughs.

Main symptoms:
- coughing fits that take your breath away
- deep, hoarse, barking cough
- cough with retching and vomiting
- the pain makes you clutch your chest when coughing
- talking is exhausting and painful
- the symptoms are worse at night or after talking or laughing and when lying down (have to sit up), and in a warm conditions

Eupatorium

Boneset – *Eupatorium perfoliatum*

Recommended:
For flu and fever with aching bones and muscles.

Main symptoms:
- caused by cold, wind and dampness
- severe aches and pains in the bones, muscles, chest; a 'beaten up' and bruised sensation
- painful cough: you have to hold your chest when coughing
- nausea and vomiting of bile
- before the fever you suffer from chills and intense thirst; sweating relieves the fever; the fever is often higher mid-morning
- throbbing headaches

Euphrasia

Eyebright – *Euphrasia officinalis*
First recommendation for a wide range of eye conditions.

Recommended:
For eye conditions and hayfever.

Main symptoms:
- dry, itching eyes; eyes feel 'gritty'
- profuse acrid tears and a runny nose with mild, bland discharge
- sensitivity to light; you have to blink constantly
- the eyes are red and you feel a burning sensation or pressure
- discharge of pus; swollen and burning eyelids
- warmth, light or wind aggravate the symptoms; you feel worse in the evenings

Ferrum phos

Iron phosphate – *Ferrum phosphoricum*
First recommendation for feverish complaints.

Recommended:
For fever, earache and nose bleeds (for nervous, delicate people, who blush easily). Often very effective in the early stages of an illness or inflamation with little or no significant symptoms.

Main symptoms:
• middle to high fever when no other significant symptoms are apparent
• bright red nose bleeds
• palpitations with a fast and soft pulse
• worse at night and better when resting

Gelsemium

Yellow Jasmine – *Gelsemium sempervirens*
First recommendation for flu.

Recommended:
For flu, fears, stage fright and nervous exhaustion.

Main symptoms:
- flu with initial chills that run up and down the spine
- head flu with a pain that rises from the back of the neck up to the eyes (sometimes accompanied by disturbed vision)
- you feel tired and exhausted; you cannot keep your eyes open
- physical and mental fatigue, feeling shivering and achy
- anticipatory fears, such as exams, interviews (possibly with trembling and diarrhoea)

Hepar sulph

Hahnemann's calcium sulphide – *Hepar sulphuris*

Recommended:
For acne, boils and other suppurations; for sore throats, coughs and earache.

Main symptoms:
- extreme sensitivity to cold; all symptoms alleviated by warmth
- irritability and anger
- suppurations have a yellow-green discharge
- intense, possibly throbbing pains and stitches, alleviated by warmth
- rough, barking, rattling cough with hoarseness
- worse in the cold

Hypericum

St. John's wort – *Hypericum perforatum*
First recommendation for injury to nerves.

Recommended:

For injuries of areas rich in sensitive nerves,
concussion of the spine and head; as a
natural antiseptic. As a cream or tincture it
speeds up the healing-process of wounds.
(*Tip:* apply a little of the tincture to mouth
ulcers and spots.)

Main symptoms:

- squashed fingers or toes
- concussion of the coccyx
- whiplash or concussion of the head
- shooting, lancing neuralgic pains
- pain after the extraction of a tooth
- puncture wounds

Ignatia

St. Ignatius Bean – *Ignatia amara*
First recommendation for emotional upsets.

Recommended:
As the main 'grief remedy' in homeopathy.

Main symptoms:
- effects of grief, sorrow, lovesickness, the loss of a loved one, homesickness, reproach, deprivation of love
- changeable moods, laughing and sobbing
- frequent sighing and yearning
- symptoms are often contradictory, e.g., you feel as if you have a lump in your throat and/or nauseous, but eating seems to help
- you feel worse after smoking, drinking coffee and in the cold

Ipecac

Ipecac-root – *Uragoga Ipecacuanha*
First recommendation for constant nausea.

Recommended:
For coughs, nausea and vomiting.

Main symptoms:
- constant nausea that is not relieved by vomiting
- the tongue is clean and without coating
- a cough with sickness and vomiting
- spasmodic cough with fear of suffocation – children become stiff and turn blue in the face during a coughing fit
- dry cough with hoarseness, but you can often hear a rattling of phlegm that refuses to budge

Kali bich

Bichromate of potash – *Kalium bichromicum*
First recommendation for sinusitis

Recommended:
For colds and sinus problems.

Main symptoms:
- thick, ropy or stringy yellow phlegm or glutinous mucus in the nose
- pressure on the root of the nose or pain in small areas of the forehead or cheekbone
- headaches, even migraine, (which may be preceded by blurred vision) from suppressed catarrh
- loss of smell, bunged up nose and sore, inflamed nostrils
- metallic cough with tough yellow phlegm
- warmth and warm steam inhalations alleviate the symptoms

Lachesis

Poison of the bushmaster snake – *Lachesis mutus*

Recommended:
For sore throats, pre-menstrual tension (PMT) and menopausal complaints.

Main symptoms:
- symptoms mostly occur on the left side of the body
- you cannot bear anything tight (around the throat or abdomen)
- sore throat, dark red in colour; swallowing is painful, warmth is intolerable
- cannot stop talking and talk very fast
- very jealous and irritable, easily envious
- hot flushes; sun and heat are unbearable
- you often feel worse after sleeping
- improves with the onset of menstruation

Ledum

Marsh tea – *Ledum palustre*

First recommendation for black eyes, bites and puncture wounds.

Recommended:

For stings and bites, puncture wounds and injuries to the eye.

Main symptoms:

- for any kind of injury where the skin is pierced: from thorns, nails, splinter, glass, etc.
- for insect stings (bee, wasp, mosquito) and bites (also ticks)
- for a black eye
- the injured area feels cold
- aggravated by warmth and movement
- cold applications (compress, etc.) bring relief

Lycopodium

Club moss – *Lycopodium clavatum*

Recommended:
For bloatedness, distension, wind.

Main symptoms:
- bloatedness, with lots of abdominal noises and rumbling; anything tight around the abdomen (waist) is extremely uncomfortable
- even the smallest amount of food makes you feel full, but soon after you feel hungry again
- strong desire for sweets
- gas and wind after eating flour-based products (pastries, etc.), garlic and onion
- symptoms may start on the right side and are often worse between 4 and 8pm

Mag phos

Phosphate of magnesia – *Magnesium phos.*
First recommendation for pains relieved by warmth.

Recommended:
For colic, stomach ache, menstrual pain, toothache, teething and sciatica (The most effective way to take the remedy is crushed in hot water and sipped.)

Main symptoms:
- spasmodic, shooting pains, eased by anything warm (hot-water bottle), tender pressure, rubbing, massage or bending double
- worse at night, in the cold and in a draft
- the pain comes and goes suddenly, or frequently changes places
- worse when you feel exhausted and worn out

Mercurius

Quicksilver – *Mercurius solubilis*
First recommendation for ulcers.

Recommended:
For toothache, earache, suppurations.

Main symptoms:
- foul breath often with a sweetish, metallic taste in the mouth
- increased saliva production, but thirsty
- the tongue is moist, swollen and has toothmarks along the sides
- inflamed, swollen gums and mouth ulcers
- toothache at night
- chronic, foetid discharge from the ear
- sticky, smelly night sweats
- you feel uncomfortable in the heat and cold

Nux vomica

Poison nut – *Nux vomica*

First recommendation for stomach upsets and hangovers.

Recommended:
For digestive disorders, nausea and retching, constipation, backache, PMT, menstrual pain, earache, disturbed sleep, hangovers.

Main symptoms:
- after-effects of rich food or food that is off, an excess of alcohol, smoking, coffee, an abuse of medical and recreational drugs, stress and a lack of sleep
- nausea with retching (you cannot vomit), food lies like a stone in the stomach
- very stressed, irritable and oversensitive
- aggravated by the cold and drafts, alleviated by the warmth

Phosphorus

Phosphorus – *Phosphorus*

Recommended:
For bleeding, coughs, hoarseness.

Main symptoms:
- bright red blood, e.g., from the nose, or after the extraction of a tooth
- easily bruised
- dry, hard cough
- hoarse, or even loss of voice
- very thirsty for cold drinks
- strong burning pains
- easily exhausted, but even a little rest or sleep refreshes
- fear of being alone, of thunderstorms, ghosts and supernatural things

Phytolacca

Poke root – *Phytolacca decandra*

Recommended:
For sore throats.

Main symptoms:
- sore throats, the throat and tonsils are dark red
- in the early stages of tonsillitis
- when you swallow, the pain extends to the ear
- the glands under the jaw and along the neck are swollen
- complaint made worse by warm drinks
- the tongue has a greasy yellow coating in the middle, the tip and sides are red
- feeling achy and bruised

Pulsatilla

Wind flower – *Pulsatilla pratensis*

Recommended:

For colds, complaints of the ear, teeth, bladder, 'female complaints', coughs, digestive problems, grief.

Main symptoms:

- symptoms are often caused by cold, dampness and grief
- a desire for gentle movement in the fresh air
- mucus (cold, cough, ear, etc.) is bland, thick and yellow or green
- digestive problems often caused by fatty, rich food, pork and ice-cream
- no thirst
- weepy and moody, a desire for company and sympathy

Rhus tox

Poison ivy – *Rhus toxicodendron*

First recommendation for strains and sprains.

Recommended:

For strains, sprains, aching joints and backache, bladder problems, colds, hoarseness.

Main symptoms:

- often caused by the cold and damp
- great restlessness and unease
- although initially painful and stiff, the condition improves with continuous gentle movement; gets worse when resting
- intense thirst
- warmth, warm applications and massages alleviate the symptoms
- the tongue often has a red tip
- aching joints when you have a cold or flu

Ruta

Common rue – *Ruta gravolens*
First recommendation for injuries to tendons and joints.

Recommended:
For injuries of the joints, tendons, ligaments, bruised bones, eye strain.

Main symptoms:
- for tennis elbow, weak joints, sore tendons, contraction of the fingers, concussion of the bones (shin)
- eye strain (computer, reading, etc.) with tired, burning eyes and neck ache
- feeling sore, stiff, bruised and weak
- worse in the damp-cold and when lying down

Sepia

Ink of the cuttlefish – *Sepia officinalis*

Recommended:

For 'female complaints', if the following symptoms are present:

Main symptoms:

- you feel you would like to leave everything behind: partner, job and family
- an aversion to your job, family and to sex
- feeling desperate and depressed; often aggressive and snappy
- feeling weak, dizzy with an inclination to perspire
- despite a feeling of weakness, symptoms improve after vigorous motion (dance, exercises)
- nausea and faintness relieved by eating
- poor circulation

Silica

Flint – *Silica*

First recommendation for opening boils and forcing out splinters.

Recommended:
For boils, abscesses and other suppurations; constipation.

Main symptoms:
- suppurations, boils, splinters in the skin
- tendency to suffer from suppurations, which heal badly and leave scars (abscess, boils, acne etc.); especially effective in the treatment of suppurations that develop slowly
- fear of needles and pins
- lack of vital heat; always cold
- tendency to sweat from the head or feet
- constipation – requires straining

Spongia

Roasted sponge – *Spongia tosta*

Recommended:
For croup-like cough.

Main symptoms:
- dry, barking cough, with wheezing and difficulty in breathing, as if you are breathing through a sponge
- coughing fits at night, shaking you out of your sleep with a suffocating sensation
- hoarseness
- you have to sit up
- you feel better after eating or drinking something warm
- you feel worse after a cold drink, before midnight and when lying down
- you may feel weak and anxious

Staphysagria

Stavesacre – *Delphinium Staphysagria*
First recommendation for styes

Recommended:
For styes, cuts and puncture wounds.

Main symptoms:
- frequently reoccurring styes, which may leave tiny hard scars after they have healed
- the after-effects of suppressed emotions, such as anger, grief and feeling criticised
- for clean cuts or puncture wounds
- the after-effects of an operation, catheter or episiotomy

S

Symphytum

Comfrey – *Symphytum officinale*

First recommendation for injuries of the bones and joints.

Recommended:

For bone injuries, broken bones, injuries to the eye. It stimulates the healing of bones.

Main symptoms:

- injured bones, joints, tendons, ligaments and muscles
- injured eye or facial bones from a blow or knock
- problems with the joints following an injury
- pressure, motion and touch make you feel worse; warmth brings relief

Veratrum

White Hellebore – *Veratrum album*

Recommended:

For diarrhoea, vomiting, stomach ache and collapse.

Main symptoms:

- feeling extremely cold, cold perspiration. You long for heat but feel no better in the warmth
- blue lips, cold tip of nose and extreme weakness
- watery diarrhoea, often accompanied by vomiting, which leaves you feeling completely exhausted
- severe spastic pain
- desire for cold water

Rescue remedy

(Drops and cream) *excellent first aid remedy*

Recommended:
For shock, injuries, burns and emergencies of any kind.

Dosage and directions:
Available in most health-food shops and pharmacies, Rescue remedy is not, strictly speaking, homeopathic, but one of the Bach Flower remedies. However, it is so effective in the treatment of the above complaints that it is a good idea always to carry a bottle around with you.

- Put 10 drops in half a glass of water and sip slowly (or apply 3–5 drops directly onto the lips or tongue). Apply the cream to the affected skin area as often as you need

USEFUL ADDRESSES

UK PHARMACIES

Helios Pharmacy has designed a homeo-pathic kit to accompany this book. This enables you to keep all the necessary remedies within easy reach both at home and when travelling. The leather wallet can contain up to 60 remedies, with a space for the book itself and can be purchased from Helios with either the 20 most important remedies (all of which are mentioned in the book) or with 40 or 60 remedies. You can add to the kit as you become more confi-dent and experienced.

For more information or to place an order, contact:

Helios Homeopathic Pharmacy
89-97 Camden Road, Tunbridge Wells,
Kent TN1 2QR. Tel: 01892
537254/536393; e-mail:
pharmacy@helios.co.uk, Web site:
www.helios.co.uk

Ainsworth Homeopathic Pharmacy
36 New Cavendish Street, London W1M
7LH. Tel: 020 7935 5330.

Goulds Homeopathic Chemist
PO Box 1019, 14 Crowndale Road,
London, NW1 1TH. Tel: 020 7388 4752

Nelson and Co. Ltd. and **Weleda** make
all the remedies mentioned. These brands
are stocked by most large chemists and
health-food stores.

Finding a homeopath in the UK

Send a SAE (24x16cm) to
The British Homeopathic Association
27a Devonshire Street, London W1N 1RJ.
Tel: 020 7935 2163

The Society of Homoeopaths
2 Artizan Road, Northampton NN1 4HU.
Tel: 01604 621400.

Sven Sommer
Mr Sommer is based in Oxford and can be
contacted by writing care of: Ebury Press,
20 Vauxhall Bridge Road, London SW1V
2SA

or by e-mailing him at
info@svensommer.com

Recommended reading

George Vithoulkas, *Medicine of the New Man*, Thorsons.

Dorothy Shepherd, *A Physician's Posy* and *The Magic of the Minimum Dose*, The C.W. Daniel Company.

Miranda Castro, *The Complete Homoeopathic Handbook*, Pan Books

Gabrielle Pinto & Murray Feldman, *Homoeopathy for Children*, The C.W. Daniel Company.

Asa Hershoff, *Homeopathic Remedies*, Avery Publishing Group.

ABOUT THE AUTHOR

Sven Sommer, Hp, MdFDH, trained in homeopathy and other complementary therapies in Germany. There he is the author of three successful books on the subject. Since 1997 he has worked and lived in Oxford. For more information, visit his website: *www.svensommer.com*